DR. BROWN

THE AMERICAN MEDICAL PROBLEM

H. DOYLE SMITH

Copyright © 2022 **AaronDenburn Publishing**

All rights reserved. No part of this publication may be reproduced, distributed, or transmitted in any form or by any means, including photocopying, recording, or other electronic or mechanical methods, without the prior written permission of the publisher, except in the case of brief quotations embodied in critical reviews and certain other noncommercial uses permitted by copyright law. For permission requests, write to the publisher, addressed "Attention: Book Rights and Permission," at the address below.

Published in the United States of America

ISBN 978-1-956741-87-2 (SC)
ISBN 978-1-956741-88-9 (Ebook)

AaronDenburn Publishing
P.O. Box 81
Dalton, OH 44618 USA
www.stellarliterary.com

Order Information and Rights Permission:

Quantity sales. Special discounts might be available on quantity purchases by corporations, associations, and others. For details, contact the publisher at the address above.

For Book Rights Adaptation and other Rights Permission. Call us at toll-free 1-888-945-8513 or send us an email at admin@stellarliterary.com.

Contents

Doctor Brown i
Introduction 1
Doctors Are People 5
The Problems 8
The System Has Engulfed a Major Portion of The Gross Domestic Product of American Business 10
    The Historical Basis 12
All Doctors and Other Personal Service Providers are Monopolies 14
    Monopoly Pricing 16
Legal consideration 18
    Malpractice Suits 19
    Protocol medicine 21
    Patents 23
The System Is Designed to Defraud Cost-Plus Pricing 24
    The Nature of Cost-plus Pricing 25
    Anybody Can Bill the System 27
Patients Are Not Required to Validate Services 28
    Anonymous Costs 29
    Quick Pay Requirement 30
    Split up Billing 32
    Part time, Too Much Income 34
    Insurance Negotiation 36
    Uncontrolled Price 38
Medicare Payments Are Used For Other Purpose Besides Health Care .. 40

- Distractions 42
  - New Doctors are Burned with Student Loans 43
  - Research and Development 44
  - Quick to specialize 46
- The Promotion of Health Care Is an Emotional Appeal, Not a Realistic One 48
  - Reliance on fear 49
- Solutions 51
- Mining the System 52
- Farming the System 53
- We Need to Invest in our Healthcare Workers 54
- More Bang for the buck 55
- Research and Development 56
  - Legal Problems Malpractice 57
  - Medical Patents 58
- Set Prices 59
- Payment to licensees only 60
- Incomplete Claims 61
- Avoid Sidetracking New Physicians 62
- Hospital Independence 63
- Summary 64

Doctor Brown

This is a study of the American medical system. Norway, according to a Facebook post has labeled this system as underdeveloped. Studies have shown that you could go to the coast of Spain, have a new knee installed and spend a week on the beach for less than the same knee surgery in America. In my own experience, I know that an emergency room visit, with 26 stitches, a tetanus shot and pain medicine cost sixty two dollars in Berlin, Germany, while nurses in Ohio estimate that the same would cost over for hundred and fifty dollars. How did this happen?

My experience with the medical infrastructure gives some light on how this developed. We need to understand that it is not the people who provide the medical services that have caused the problem, but the system itself. It has several problems that should be addressed. And there are solutions that would rectify the situation if we have a willingness to deal with these problems, instead of bemoaning the difficulties that we face. Each of these statements will be dealt with in this study,

Introduction

This is a study of the medical system in the United States. It has grown through time from an inadequately financed hit or miss business to a major part of our economy. The best way to start is to look at how the system has grown over the last 85 years to the situation we find ourselves in today. Since I have been involved in this industry as much as I have, the best way to introduce the subject is to follow my experience in it.

I grew up in a small town in the mountains of North Carolina. We grew our own food, took our corn to the mill and allowed the miller to keep a portion of that cornmeal as a payment for grinding it. This was before the Second World War, and there was little cash available to pay for anything, much less the doctor when we were sick. The idea of a hospital was talked about but there was no money available to build one. Our only medical help was the doctor and it had to be in our home.

The stories told about Doctor Brown were a conversation starter on any occasion. His driving was atrocious. When Doctor Brown was seen coming toward you, you got out of his way. There were two reasons for this. First you were terrified that you would be in an accident, and second you knew Doc Brown was on his way to a patient. If you were sick at later time you wanted to know that Doc Brown could get to our house to take care of you.

It was a simple life then. One of my jobs, until I went to college, was to hoe the corn and the rest of the garden. We kept a pig every year and a cow supplied us the milk that we needed. Even though we were fairly affluent - my mother was a teacher and my father worked at the factory — there was little cash available. Most of the people in the area paid their doctor bills with chickens or corn, so Doctor Brown was not the wealthiest man in town.

This situation was not in the best interest of anyone. The medical profession determined that something had to be done and the doctors founded the insurance companies Blue Cross and 2

Blue shield. This allowed people to pay monthly payments that were invested, and receive health care when they needed it. The doctors were able to receive the monies that they needed to live on.

I went to college in Tucson, Arizona. There the hospitals were more affluent. During this time Medicare was instituted, and medicine was put on a more secure financial basis. Part of the credit for this was such foundations as the Duke Foundation. Other foundations and agencies helped, and the hospital throughout the country were now supported well enough that they were financially secure. The hunger of the earlier years was not forgotten. The hospitals now could make a profit, but the history of poverty was not forgotten, and the efforts to be profitable did not stop.

I have mentioned the profit of the hospitals. No business, no matter what they say, can be non-profit. If it does not make a profit it will be unable to pay bills, salary, or new equipment. The idea of something being non- profit sounds much better than the idea of a hospital being non-proprietary, but the real meaning of non-profit was that it was not owned by a person. It also reflects the idea that a hospital should not pay taxes, no matter how profitable it is. This freedom from taxation allowed investors to look toward hospitals as a sound investment, and also allowed the hospitals to invest their profit and compete with other businesses on a favorable basis.

As time went by, the town I lived in decided to try to build a hospital and with grants from foundations and a widower named Pardee, the town succeeded in building the Margaret Pardee Memorial Hospital. This is not the only hospital funded in this way. Cornelius

Aultman's widow and daughter had done the same in Canton, Ohio in the 1890's, and there are more examples throughout the country.

Heath care improved over time. Most people found that health services were better as time went on and new procedures and funding made it easier to deal with sickness. I remember that I lost many teeth due to abscesses because root canals weren't available. Now root canals are routine.

I went to college in the 1950's and became an accountant. Several years later I became the hospital controller at my local hospital during the transition from manual to computer operations in the health industry. One of my obligations was to prepare the Medicare report.

I had married a physical therapist, whom I had met at school in Tucson. She had worked there before we returned to my hometown. She was dedicated to her job. This meant was not able to find the time to make our maniage work, but I remained married to her for twenty-five years. During those years I was part of the medical community in the town, and got to know the health care professionals well.

They are all good people, but the system created problems that enticed them to do things that were not in the best interests of the patients. For example, there was money available now, and often the practice gave the doctor enough money for all his needs in three days of work, so the office would be closed on Thursday and Friday, or two other days in the week. This was a reduction of professional services of forty percent - not because the doctor wasn't involved in his practice, but because the system allowed it.

Another consideration that could be seen was that doctors and laymen are born equal, but progress, over time, until they are very different. When doctors are sued for malpractice these terms are confused. A jury of one's peers, as specified in the Magna Carta, is not the same as a jury of one's equals. We are all born equal, but we are not peers when a doctor has to spend as much as thirty-five years to become qualified and the layman may not attend school at all. A doctor has every reason to protect his investment in becoming a doctor. I will discuss these considerations separately.

In the years since that time, I have been aware of the medical profession, and have some ideas about how it works or doesn't work today

The system was developed over time and each other time a change occurred the change was not coordinated with the prior element of the system. Now we have a system that is full of problems, most of difficulties just grew, like Topsy

Doctors Are People

As a member of the medical community in our town, I attended many parties and meetings with the doctors. At one such meeting I heard a doctor comment on another doctor. He said that he would never refer any patients to him because, 'He was a butcher." He didn't state his opinion of the other doctor in public because he would have caused the other doctor to be at risk of losing his license and if he did that to the other doctor; he could be at risk for another doctor doing something like it to him.

Doctors have great respect for the effort any doctor has invested in his profession. That effort includes grammar and high school, college, medical school, internship and residency. It is not inconceivable that he would be thirty-five years old before he would be licensed to practice.

Another doctor refened me to a urologist. The urologist wondered why he had referred me. My signs were within the normal range and there was no reason that I would need he services. My doctor knew he needed the work, and had referred me to him to help him get started.

Another doctor, a retired dentist, when asked for a reference to another dentist referred me to a young dentist because the new dentist needed the work. When I found that the dentist was not as competent as I would like, the damage to my teeth was irreversible.

Doctors are proud of their profession. There is a comment that the difference between God and a doctor is that God doesn't think He's a doctor. When you invest as much time and effort in becoming a doctor to help people, you should be proud, and doctors do help people.

When doctors are well paid, they like to use what they have been paid for those things that make life enjoyable, but they try to protect their prosperity from people's envy. There is a road on the map of my county that is not easy to find. Using the map, I chose to find that road. There were two big rhododendron bushes on each side of this dirt road, and the road was not visible, seemingly a part of the bushes. When I turned into this road and crossed a hill, I saw on one side of the road a four-story house about one hundred feet long with horse pastures on three sides of the house. Below the road on the other side was a chateau beautifully landscaped. Both these houses, I found out, were houses owned and used by doctors.

Doctors, like all people, are hurt when people accuse them of what they feel they are not guilty of. I wrote a book about the fact that doctors who earn in three days what they need to live on are not likely to keep the office open on Thursday. This doctor did close his office on Thursday, and felt that I was attacking him personally. This is normal human behavior. He personalized the general circumstances, taking my book as an attack on him.

A group of doctors in my town had the means to provide all that one of them needed to fund a clinic in Africa. Other doctors volunteered to work on weekends to take care of patients for free in the charity REMOTE AREA MEDICAL in Knoxville, Tennessee. These doctors provided medical services that were not available to these people otherwise. They had the where-with all to provide services for free. These services were not available to the general public.

With such a long preparatory period in a doctor's profession it is not surprising that doctors have large amounts of educational debt. The early period of a doctor's practice are usually given over to repaying that debt.

This discussion makes it clear that doctors are people just like the rest of us, but they have a specialized knowledge of a particular subject that is helpful to most people.

The Problems

It would be nice if the problems that plague our health care could be solved by a short incantation, but they cannot. Just as the problems are complex, the solutions must be complex. Taking each problem in turn makes the solution of the individual problems less a challenge, but there cannot be one overall panacea.

A SUMMARY OF WHAT'S TO COME

Let's list some of the problems that are a part of the system. The list will be long, and each will have to be addressed separately

1. The system has engulfed approximately seventeen percent of the gross domestic product of American business
2. All doctors and other personal service providers are monopolies.
3. Legal problems.
    a. Patents
    b. Malpractice suits
    c. Protocol medicine
4. System designed to defraud
    a. Cost plus calculation
    b. Anybody can bill the system

     i. There is no list of eligible recipients
     ii. Patients are not required to validate the services
     iii. Anonymous cost
     iv. Quick pay requirements
     v. Split up billing
     vi. Part time
     vii. Insurance negotiation
     viii. Uncontrolled price
5. Medical payments are used for other purposes besides health care
6. Distractions
    a. New doctors are burned with student loans
    b. R&D
    c. Quick Specialize
7. The promotion of health care is an emotional appeal, not a realistic one
    a. Reliance on fear
    b. Indiscriminate advertising

The System Has Engulfed a Major Portion of The Gross Domestic Product of American Business

There are two factors that are part of what is needed to understand this problem.

The first factor is the role that efficiency plays in this process.

There are three stages in any endeavor. The first stage is the set-up when the things that are needed are accumulated. The second stage is when the endeavor produces the product. The third stage comes when the product is no more needed. This is the stage when what has been used must be disposed of.

The second factor is that concentration of business endeavors takes place over time, and this concentration leads to people being left out of the economy. This results in a situation where people fight to destroy what is giving them a problem and subsequently we end up with anarchy.

The first of these factors is a study in mechanics. It takes time to become efficient in any endeavor, and there is no value in this process. No matter how efficient a process is, if it is not used to produce a usable product the effort of setting it up is wasted, so there is no value in this stage. However, it is an essential element of any business.

I had an economics professor who was skilled at teaching the subject. I had noticed that she had never discussed the nature of "demand" and asked for her help in understanding it. Her response startled me, "We have to stop somewhere."

My challenge meant that the years she had spent becoming efficient were her investment (set-up) in a profession. My challenge would have meant that she would have to go back to that study, and her current stability in her profession would have to be redone. This is typical of most people. New ideas and changes mean that the efforts they have made in the past are being devalued and more investment in time and effort will be needed for the investment to be profitable.

The second factor mentioned above happens because the set-up process mentioned above becomes more efficient over time, and those who would like to enter the field must compete with a business process that has already become efficient. There is little reason for me to compete with Amazon, if Amazon has already conquered the field of on-line shopping. While I am spinning my wheels trying to get started, Amazon is continuing to serve the people that I would have to rely on if I were to get my business started. The efficiency of the business in place will always overcome the start-up company that must, by nature be less efficient and therefore more costly. As monopolies arise the people at the top prosper and the other people find they have less and less with which to accomplish their objectives.

The Historical Basis

That the cycle mentioned above is a real cycle can to be demonstrated by a reference to history. After the Civil War the productivity of the American manufacturer became legendary. Prior to that war, America was principally an agricultural nation providing farm produce to older nations that had less agricultural land, and needed the food, (wheat) clothing (cotton) and other basic resources that America could provide.

The organizational methods that the military developed during the process of the war enabled the entrepreneurs to establish their businesses on a sound basis. In fact the efficiency of the new methods of business made the productive capacity of the Americans of that day more than similar production anywhere else in history. But the efficiency involved did not reach the average laborer and those people who had to work for the entrepreneurs, often had to do without what they needed to live well. Accidents on the job were not treated; sickness meant no income, and the efficiency of the entrepreneurs did not reach the average individual.

As a result over time these workers, when they had the opportunity, voiced their concerns, and in the early twentieth century the government outlawed monopoly, (The Sherman Anti-Tmst Act and others) and labor unions were formed. The lack of customers when all people had all they wanted meant that eventually the business could not sustain their productivity, and the Great Depression followed. The anarchy that was an everyday life to the hoboes and out-of-work people during that period lasted until the Second World War demanded the production that these people could provide.

We have only been a country for a few hundred years. That this cycle is recurrent is best indicated by the history of China. There the cycle has recurred consistently over a period of at least three thousand years.

If you wonder where in this cycle we are now, you will notice that many people are left out of the economy by consolidation of the means of earning a living. Others are accumulating those means and denying them to those who could use them. The value of each person as a part of the whole society is based on the objective that that person has chosen to accomplish for the good of all. Those resources that are needed to accomplish such objectives are in the hands of people who cannot use them because they are too many resources for the objectives that the owners can accomplish. Bill Gates has a great deal of wealth and has chosen to use it for the benefit of otherwise unattainable objectives, such as elimination of malaria, but other wealthy people simply allow the resources they control to not be used.

The poorest people who exist are those people who have all the resources they can ever accumulate, but have no way or plan to use them. Let me say this clearly. It is not the payment for healthcare that matters. It is the healthcare services themselves.

All Doctors and Other Personal Service Providers are Monopolies

There is another factor that applies to medicine; ANY PERSONAL SERVICE BUSINESS IS A MONOPOLY.

I do not approach several doctors to determine which is the cheapest. My relationship with a doctor, like my relationship with a lawyer, or Tax preparer is determined by whether I trust the doctor, and that relationship is exclusive. As a result, if you want to use the doctor's services you pay what is required. As a result the prices the doctor charges are not restricted by competition, or by any other mechanism.

When this problem was noted during the Great Depression, it was found in the fact that electric wires to homes could not allow competition. Each company would have its separate wire on poles through the city or there would be a major number of wires everywhere. The electric companies were declared to be monopolies (utilities) and each was given a certain area where they would provide services. In exchange, the monopolies were limited in the profit they could make. As a result, there were not an excessive number of electrical wires to deal with and the monopolies had a sufficient income. They could not overcharge.

This understanding has not been noted in the medical profession. Because the fact that they are monopolies has not been noticed, various methods have been allowed that maximize the profits of the profession. In competitive situations that has been limited by the idea that if I don't buy it here, I can go to another doctor. Even though second opinions are often asked for, most people do not feel right to spread their personal information to too many people and as long as the doctor is trusted, that doctor will be the one the person goes to.

This is the basis of monopoly. Because the doctor has this monopoly he is free to charge whatever will be paid. In this case, Medicare has allowed the doctors to receive the rewards for a major part of the gross domestic product in this monopolistic situation.

Monopoly Pricing

Monopolies are able to price their services without regard to competitive considerations. As a result, there is little reason to keep prices low. As I noted above, we have a problem with patents. Synthroid and insulin are patented medicines that are essential to the health of many people. Because of patent rights they can only be manufactured by the company with the patent. If the patents were made permanent, but available to all qualified manufacturers with set royalties, the cost of these products could be controlled. Another consideration that could be seen was that doctors and laymen are born equal, but progress, over time, until they are very different. When doctors are sued for malpractice these terms are confused.

All hospitals are monopolies. In any personal service business, the relationship between the provider and the customer is a monopoly. I do not take my tax information to every CPA in town to find out what his price is before I give him my personal information. I determine who I trust and deal only with that person. The same rule holds true for lawyers and physicians. This means that I am dependent on the good faith of my personal service provider, and though I may choose to get a second opinion, the question is whether I trust my doctor or not, not that I want to compare prices.

This means that I end up paying what the doctor charges, or if I am using insurance, the company pays what the doctor charges. Unfortunately, the insurance company is in a position to negotiate payment. When the doctor negotiates with an insurance company, and accepts a lesser price, he does not give you the same price as he has accepted from the negotiation. In fact, the amount that is reduced for the insurance company will be raised for others so that neither the doctor nor the insurance company will lose.

The fact that the doctor's services are monopolies means that the laws of economics do not apply to those services. Unfortunately, most people who have some economic background try to use economics as a basis for analyzing medical services.

Doctors who have been admitted to practice have another lure that reduces health services. A doctor who was a researcher, studying cases that were rare affecting less than one percent of the population — found that he had cancer. He opened an office in our town and in two years earned enough to fund his family's security before he died. Had he been providing those services instead of researching a rare disease, the health care he provided would have been a real help in reducing the problems of his patients.

Legal consideration

We have already noted that juries in cases involving physicians are made up of "equal" citizens. Some become Doctors and are the peers of other doctors, but the word peer is not the same as what we are born with. We read in the Declaration of Independence that all people are created equal, but they develop differently. . A jury of one's peers, as specified in the Magna Carta, is not the same as a jury of one's equals. We are all born equal, but we are not peers when a doctor has to spend as much as thirty-five years to become qualified and the layman may not attend school at all.

The expectation that litigation will find the doctor at fault whether he has done his best or not makes malpractice cases a real threat to physicians. Since, usually, no one on the jury is a peer of the physician, there is little likelihood of a favorable result from such a suit as far as the doctor can expect. Although there should be at least one member of the jury who is a peer of the plaintiff, so should there be a member of the jury who is the peer of the doctor.

Malpractice Suits

I am going to repeat what I just wrote. It's important. We have already noted that juries in cases involving physicians are made up of "equal" citizens. We read in the Declaration of Independence that all people are created equal, but they develop differently. Some become Doctors and are the peers of other doctors, but the word peer is not the same condition that we are we are born with.

The expectation that litigation will find the doctor at fault whether he has done his best or not makes malpractice cases areal threat to physicians. Since, usually, no one on the jury is a peer of the physician, there is little likelihood of a favorable result from such a suit as far as the doctor can expect. Although there should be at least one member of the jury who is a peer of the plaintiff, so should there be a member of the jury who is the peerof the doctor.

This involves two different problems. The first is the fear of litigation. I had a growth on my gums. The surgeon froze it off. When we were getting ready for the procedure, he suggested that he take a sample for a biopsy. I asked him what he would be able to do if the biopsy came back positive. 1--1e admitted that there was little he could do, so I suggested that we omit the biopsy. The cost of the removal was $185. The cost of the same procedure with the biopsy he estimated to be $845. The biopsy would have been a mitigating circumstance if we had been going to court, so if I had not talked with him about omitting it, it would have cost me $660 for no result. I had to convince this doctor that I would not sue. Had he not understood that, he would have insisted that that I accept the biopsy.

Medical malpractice suits are a double threat to physicians. There is a significant threat that the litigation will require a penalty based on a judgment. This requirement for payment is significant, but the real threat is that the doctor's reputation would preclude the trust of his patients. If patients will not use the doctor's services, he cannot remain in practice.

Protocol medicine

A second problem involves using procedures that have been litigated before, instead of diagnoses to treat patients. A doctor who was to treat my back saw the same x-ray that I saw. It showed a piece of bone loose next to my spine. The doctor said that he would treat the back "conservatively" and prescribed 18 physical therapy treatments. By the twelfth treatment I was in constant pain, but the doctor could not be sued because he was following the protocol for that problem. The use of procedural treatments meant that he could not be sued, even though the diagnosis required a different treatment.

The problem here is not for the doctor, but for the patient. If the diagnosis contradicts the protocol, the patient will never receive adequate medical treatment. We have already noted that juries in cases involving physicians are made up of "equal" citizens. We read in the Declaration of Independence that all people are created equal, but they develop differently. Some become Doctors and are the peers of other doctors, but the word peer is not the same as what we are born with. .

The expectation that litigation will find the doctor at fault whether he has done his best or not makes malpractice cases a real threat to physicians. Since, usually, no one on the jury is a peer of the physician, there is little likelihood of a favorable result from such a suit as far as the doctor can expect. Although there should be at least one member of the jury who is a peer of the plaintiff, so should there be a member of the jury who is the peer of the doctor.

Patents

New medicines are patented, giving the inventor a monopoly on the product invented for a certain period of time to reward his initiative in formulating the new product, procedure, or idea. This is an incentive to encourage invention and works well in increasing the knowledge, and ease with which we develop better procedures in our daily lives. These patents encourage development of the medicines that will help the patients. Without such encouragement, some important medicines would have never been discovered.

This provides the discoverer the right to exclusive production and distribution of the new medicine for a period of time and encourages research. This has developed many new medicines over time.

However, some of these patents cover medicines that are needed by people to survive. Insulin and Synthroid are essential medicines for those people who have the diseases that they are intended to treat.

The monopoly that the patent gives increases the price that the user must pay to live. Such patents need to be made perpetual, but must be licensed to any manufacturer who can prove that the product can be produced safely. This possible solution would both maintain the incentive to research, and allow competition to keep the costs in a reasonable range.

The System Is Designed to Defraud Cost-Plus Pricing

This section will be discussed again later. I prepared three Medicare reports as a hospital controller. These reports determine what the government will pay the hospital for its services. It has provided these funds on a cost-plus basis. Any contractor knows that if he has the right to determine the costs and the payment will be made by someone else, he can buy expensive parts and justify those parts by selling the idea that they are needed. A contractor has the option of selling a doctor a ten-cent scalpel or a state-of-the-art electronic knife. Since the cost will be paid by Medicare and the doctor will have far better equipment, there is no incentive to reduce costs.

Costs are arbitrary figures. In a study I performed for a congressman some years ago, three hospitals in western North Carolina found a way to increase the housekeeping costs on the Medicare report by forty percent by changing the way they are calculated. That increase occurred even though none of these hospitals increased the size of the facility, or the staff of that facility. It is impossible to imagine any doctor not choosing the more expensive option.

The Nature of Cost-plus Pricing

I had a car accident and took my car to the dealer to be repaired. He estimated my cost of repair at $1800, but added, "I do not know what else we may need to do once we get into it. I took it to another shop, where they investigated what was needed and came up with an estimate of $9,000. I chose the estimate of $9,000. The price was set, and I knew that the amount I would pay was $9,000. Had I chosen the lesser figure the dealer would have found that this would be needed, and that would be needed, and by the time it was done I might have had to pay more than the $9,000. The first estimate was cost plus, the second was firm.

I rehabilitated an old house. At the start I told the carpenter that I wanted to sell it for $35,000. Because the price was not firm, he offered improvements that ended up costing $33,000 and with other costs involved I would have paid out more than the sales price of the house. I lost my shirt.

In both these cases, I found that the difference between a cost-plus contract and a firm one is the difference between profitability and loss.

Medicare is a cost-plus contract. The professional uses the methods and supplies and Medicare must pay what those costs require, usually without time or resources to verify that the costs are real or warranted. This is done by means of the Medicare report that is required once each year. I prepared three of these reports.. It was a typical adjustment of the costs that increased income to the provider without one additional justification.

Anybody Can Bill the System

A different problem arises when the invoices are to be paid without verifying that the provider is qualified to bill Medicare. There is no list of eligible recipients. Anyone who knows the process involved in billing Medicare has the ability to make a bill that would be accepted by the agency. Congress has made it necessary to pay such a bill within a certain number of days. The fraudulent billing has to be accepted by Medicare, and paid. There have been cases reported in the newspapers of this happening frequently.

The rush to payment requires that any bill presented to Medicare can only be audited after the payment has been made. In this case the payment was made to a fictitious entity that disappears before the audit has occurred. It would be a simple thing to require that license number and licensing agency for each provider on each invoice and consider it incomplete and not ready for payment without these identifications. The payment would go to the address of the licensee.

By requiring that only those who are licensed receive payment, the government can be assured that the business they are paying will be there when the payment is audited and discrepancies found. For those health care needs that are provided by non-licensed vendors, the licensed healthcare professional will bill Medicare and pay the vendor.

Patients Are Not Required to Validate Services

As an auditor I always wanted to know what the consideration of payment of invoices was. In other words, I wanted to know what the company was buying. The current process of billing for Medicare charges leaves the patient out of the loop. A bill for services is submitted to Medicare. No provision for the patient to question whether the bill was valid or not. By leaving the patient out of the loop, whatever knowledge the patient has as to whether the bill should be paid or not is lost.

The patient is the only one who can say that a given procedure was used in their case, and this deficiency makes any invoice questionable. While my wife was in the hospital, her oncologist came by and said hello. Later she found that the hello had cost Medicare $150. There was nothing medical about the visit but Medicare paid for his visit. The patient is the only person who has been involved in the procedure. By paying the bill without having the patient review it, the Medicare agency is flying blind in verifying wheather the procedures were provided or not.

Anonymous Costs

There is another limitation to auditing for Medicare auditors. My wife had knee replacement surgery. We received a copy of the bill from the hospital and saw that it consisted of line after line with these descriptions, "Hospital miscellaneous - $8.90, Hospital miscellaneous - $15,000.00." There was no way in any conceivable process to audit such a bill. That hospital has now been put out of business by the monopolistic health structure in this area, but the practice of hiding the nature of the services by poor billing probably is continuing.

There is a difference in cost between Clopidigrel and Plavix. They are the same medicine, but the doctor will refer to Clopidigrel as Plavix. The invoice submitted to Medicare for payment should identify the precise medicine used. By identifying Clopidigrel as Plavix the price of the item purchased is overstated.

Every medicine and procedure should be identified by name, dose and supplier. By calling everything "hospital miscellaneous," the health professional has succeeded in hiding the source, type and nature of the charge.

Of course, there will be certain items that cannot be identified, but they should not amount to more than a small part of the charges. There is little value in determining that a cost of a supply would only vary by a dollar or so when the agency is dealing with millions.

Quick Pay Requirement

Associated with the section above, there is another problem. By law, the payment process is so quick that the submission of bills cannot be properly audited before the bills are paid. This is a loophole that has allowed many scams. A dummy operation is set up, and the operation prepares bills for non-existent patients. To obey the law these bills must be paid within a certain amount of time. There is no time to audit them and they are paid before the auditor has a chance to find that they are fraudulent. Of course, the billing agency has closed his business before the auditor finds that it is fraudulent, and the payment can never be recovered.

Governmental agencies are notorious for slow payment. Work done by a dairy equipment company for Ohio State University was billed and the company estimated that the payment would be no earlier than two months from the billing. Partly this is because governmental agencies are aware that they are responsible for not wasting the people's money and want to assure that the appearance that they did never surfaces. They do not want to have to deal with the fallout from wasted money.

The same idea was in effect with health care. Unfortunately, Health care professionals do not want to have their receivables take that long. Congress, to help these professionals, passed a law that says that health care invoices to Medicare would be paid within a much shorter period that is usual for the typical governmental agency. This would have been no problem if the payee was known and a stable business, but it opened the doors to a means that would allow manipulation of the system by fly by night operators. It would have been no problem if Medicare could be assured that the billing provider could be located after the payment was made but there is no assurance that the company will still be there in many cases.

This would be no problem if the only people able to be paid by Medicare were licensed health care providers, as we have discussed above. By requiring that the payment be to only those who have proven that they are providing proper health care, and have proven their ability to do the job this loophole would be closed. Payment could be both prompt and auditable since the supplier can be identified for audit later.

Split up Billing

I went to a doctor with back pain. In dealing with this doctor, a problem became evident. He prescribed physical therapy, a department of the complex where he practiced. This department was a separate corporation from the doctor, and billed its services separately. In fact, this complex included MRI, surgery room, x-ray, and several other departments, each of which billed its charges separately. By making each charge separately, the complex could effectively hide the total cost of each case.

Later he prescribed physical therapy treatments, MRI imaging, and pain management. Each of these was handled by a separate business and billed separately. I had one problem, but the billing was split up between each of the different parts of the business since each was a separate business. The true cost of my health care was split up so that there could never be an accurate total.

This usually remedied in another industry, construction, by having a general contractor and subcontractors to accomplish the construction. The general contractor deals with the buyer, and the subcontractors deal only with the general contractor.

In the case of health care, the same procedure would enable the agency to determine the total cost of the treatment and determine what those total costs should be. As it is now, the totals for different treatments are hidden. By using the same process that would enable these costs to be determined. This would be valuable if the prescribing doctor could establish a job as separate from all other jobs, pay the radiologist, physical therapist, occupational therapist and any other technician that might be required, then billing the total amount for the treatment.

Part time, Too Much Income

I have mentioned above the fact that a doctor who earns enough in three days to meet all of his needs will be uninterested in working the rest of the week, meaning that health services in this case are reduced by forty percent. When people earn too much money they have a tendency to not work hard. There is no real incentive in keeping the office open when there are many other things that attract the health provider's interest. This is a greater problem than most because people tend to think that more money increases more production. This does not happen in a monopoly. The monopolist can charge whatever he chooses and the buyer of his product must pay or do without.

We have a problem in this country with monopolies. Microsoft is the only provider of computer internet infrastructure. Google is the only real alternative for internet access. Amazon is the only provider of internet sales. The result of this concentration is that Macy's employees are without work, Penny's is no longer capable of providing cheap but quality clothing, and the monopoly companies can charge whatever price they can get. If you want the product you pay the monopolist's price. If you cannot pay that price you can do without.

The clinics that the charity, Remote Area Medical, provides illustrate the need for medical services that are unmet, because of this out of balance economy. If the Doctors kept their offices available full time many of these health problems could be dealt with, but the way the system works, many of these people who need health must do without

Doctors who want to be part of the solution of this problem should show that they are working at a rate of at least 1800 hours a year. There are 2080 hours in a year in total. With vacation and holidays, - totaling 15 days, or 120 hours leaving 1960 hours — there are still twenty days available to relax. If they are not working at such a rate they should not participate in Medicare. Professional education and vacations should be allowed as part of this rate, but health care providers should be willing to provide health care when it is needed.

Insurance Negotiation

Blue Cross and Blue shield placed the medical industry on a sound basis. Doctors were paid regularly and patients were able to pay for health services in a way that they could afford. But all good things have their dark side. Insurance is a profitable industry. The accumulated premiums can be invested and the investment provides interest income without work. To pay out claims reduces the income that the insurance company can earn. There is an inbom aversion then to paying out claims.

Since it is not good business for insurance companies to pay out claims, they usually try to limit the pay-out as much as possible. Insurance companies then find it is good business to negotiate lower payouts. Since the doctor is dependent on an insurance company for most of his income, he is prone to accept less from an insurance company than he would accept from the patient directly.

In one case, the doctor asked for insurance information from a patient, and commented that the insurance company would settle the claim for $800. When the patient decided to pay the bill in cash, the doctor billed hem $1500. The situation precluded the patient from paying the bill himself, and locked the doctor into a system that required insurance. Usually if you pay in cash it should be less than what would be expected from an insurance company, but the strength of the insurance industry precludes such a result

Cost plus billing should be replaced with firm price billing as we have seen above. The same requirement should mean that the insurance industry would pay the firm price as well.

Uncontrolled Price

Both cost plus pricing and insurance negotiation place the patient at a disadvantage. The money that must be spent for health care must be accumulated, and this accumulation helps the patient by making the money needed available when that money is needed. For this reason insurance is essential, but over accumulation and negotiated prices make health care secondary to financial concerns. By allowing negotiation and not a firm price for each procedure the cost of health care exceeds the value of health care. The difference must be made up, usually by charging more from the patient or the government. Since the security of the health care industry is no longer in question, we need to assure that the methods used in making the industry secure are not used the mine the government.

Mining and farming are two different ways to look at any industry. Miners find a lode of minerals that have value and mine it until there is no mineral left. Ghost towns of the West are the result of such mining. Men can no longer live there since there is nothing of value left. Farming on the other hand requires that the fann be maintained for perpetual use.

The insurance industry has the option of being a farming operation or a mining operation. Workman's compensation in Ohio has taken the choice of farming the funds that are required to provide health care to those who are injured on the job. As much effort of the agency is spent on preventing injuries as is spent on treating those who are injured. This means that there are fewer injuries to treat and a saving of money that would otherwise need to be spent. The option of insurance companies to use their funds to prevent illness, rather than treat illnesses after they occur should be encouraged.

Medicare Payments Are Used For Other Purpose Besides Health Care

Aultman Hospital In Canton, Ohio, and other hospitals have other businesses that are favored by the fact that hospitals are nonprofit. Being exempt from taxes allows the hospital to compete favorably with other businesses that do have to pay taxes. In Canton, many doctors and other health care professionals rent their offices from the hospital. These offices are not part of the hospital, and if these renters were to rent from someone else, they would have the same offices, but with the hospital not paying taxes the rent would need to be more expensive. By using the tax exempt status to avoid paying taxes, the hospital is in a clearly advantageous position.

More critically several hospitals nearby have their own health insurance business. This is clearly a conflict of interest. A friend recommended a doctor to me who had done a good job with his back surgery. I attempted to get an appointment with him, however, my physician informed me that he could not take my case because I had Anthem insurance. He said, "They don't want another insurance company getting into their hospital.

Dealing in unrelated businesses, and favoring their own insurance companies are problems that favor hospitals greatly. To deal with this flagrant favoritism requires that the field be leveled. That can be most easily done by requiring that any governing board member of the hospital relinquish any governing power over any other business.

Distractions

There are many distractions that affect our health care industry. I will discuss three. Doctors are burdened with student debt, and have to charge as much as they can. Since this is born in the early stages of their career, they are distracted from their practice in order to keep their finances in order.

Too much of the health care industry is dedicated to research and development. As I discussed earlier the set up stage of any endeavor is worthless unless it is put into production. This research and development is part of the set up stage of medical practice, and unless it develops a good process for better health it does not have real value.

Again, it is nice to be specialist, and to be considered an expert in your field, But a person who specializes can only be useful if that special case exists. Too much specialization removes the physician from caring for the everyday ordinary patient.

New Doctors are Burned with Student Loans

A doctor, to Qualify as a doctor, must spend more years in becoming qualified to practice than almost any other profession. This means that his student costs are higher than most other professions. Because they are incuned prior to his being licensed to practice the cost of this setup is difficult to recover and especially difficult since income in such a case is slow to develop. This means that the doctor is pushed to recover his costs of education and this cost recovery takes a toll on his early career.

This distraction is easy for people to understand, so it is a good thing to look for a solution.

One solution is for the government to buy all the doctor's educational debt, and amortize that debt over a twenty year period. Since the purpose of the debt is to allow him to serve the public a second part of this amortization would be forgiveness of the debt at the same rate, if the doctor showed that he worked at a rate of 1800 hours per year. This provides a means for the doctor to eliminate his student debt by providing health care services in a reasonable manner.

Research and Development

When Jesus talked about the lost sheep, and the shepherd searching for him, He made it clear that the ninety and nine sheep were safely in the foal. We need to consider this ratio when we talk about research and development. Those people who need health care should not suffer because too much is put into our research and development. A newly licensed physician should not be involved in research or development until he has worked as a general practitioner for a reasonable time, say two years. If he does, he needs to be deprived of the forgiveness that was mentioned in the section above.

The use of research is to discover how to deal with problems that are prevalent in the medical field currently. Usually, the efforts of research that I have seen involve problems that do not affect a majority of patients. One is focused on cleft palate. The same people who have cleft palates are not isolated. These people have other more serious problems, and the effort for alleviating these problems should not be limited to one part of it.

Since we are talking about the government's efforts to deal with medical problems, it is important to note that private funds are not bound by the need to provide extensive and comprehensive care to the public at large. This need does not limit the efforts of private individuals to work toward objectives that they have identified, but wherever research has removed health care provision that would be available to the general public for diseases that need to be dealt with, this sidetrack is a problem.

Quick to specialize

Specialists concentrate on only one disease. This means that when there is no patient with this disease they are usually not occupied in practicing medicine. The training and work that they have spent in becoming physicians is not being used. Since specialists can charge more than other physicians, physicians are subject to the temptation to go into the specialties quickly. Certain specialists, such as pediatricians and gynecologists, are active more than others. These specialties are not a problem, but some others enable the physician to keep his office open only a few days a week.

Several of the problems mentioned above, as well as this problem, can be alleviated by making it a rule that if a physician fails to maintain a working environment for enough hours in a year. Medicare reimbursement should be denied to physicians who work, including vacations, holidays, professional education and actual time in the office at a rate of less than a certain number of hours a yearwill not be allowed to participate in Medicare. There are 2080 hours in a year if a forty hour week is expected. If physicians work at a rate that would provide nearly that number of hours in a year, there would be no problem. Specialists could practice as general practitioners when ther is no need for their specialties.

Of course practitioners who have in in practice for a certain number of years would be exempt from this requirement. Additionally physicians who specialize before they have practiced in general medicine or specialties that have a great number of cases should be denied Medicare reimbursement.

This solution could be extended to student loan forgiveness as well.

The Promotion of Health Care Is an Emotional Appeal, Not a Realistic One

The trials of health care professionals, such as Dr. Brown, have made the emotional effort to reward health care professional an endemic problem with health care. When these problems were solved, we did not stop at that point and have gone far beyond what was needed to deal with that problem. It is time we acknowledged that we need to use real facts to rule our efforts to deal with the problems of health care. The people who do the work to keep us healthy are not to blame for this situation, but our system of rewarding health care workers needs to be understood.

Reliance on fear

Additionally, we need to understand that we do not need to be afraid of the lack of health care. Humankind has existed for many years without the need for a doctor at hand for every cough, sneeze, or stuffy nose. We have developed a health care system that provides real relief for real diseases, and those diseases should be cared for, but the trip to the doctor because you scraped your knee is hardly in the nature of a real health care crisis.

Advertisers have worked hard to get people to become patients. This is not in the best interests of Americans, and we need to take care of our own health to the extent we can.

Winston Churchill is quoted as saying that free speech is messy, but we need it, like pain, to know what is going on. Our emotional nature tends to feel that, like free speech, is messy and have chosen to treat pain by avoiding it as much as possible This treating the symptom is an aid to medical merchants who want to mine the system. Instead of tolerating the pain until we treat the problem, we treat the pain. Of course the problem that caused the pain in the first place is still there and the pain returns. Our addiction to painkillers can be seen in the number of over the counter pain killers are on the shelves of pharmacies. Tylenol, Advil, Oxycontin and other painkillers have no other purpose than to reduce the pain without treating the problem that caused the pain. This is extremely helpful to those who would mine the system, extracting every dollar by what amounts to extortion.

Christians are taught not to be afraid. Fear allows the things we fear to rule our lives. By encouraging fear in the advertising that medical advertisers use these practitioners attempt to force patients to use their product whether they need it or not. This is extortion.

Solutions

The Problems we have discussed are interlocking. Sometimes one solution will cover several of these problems. Other problems require more thought.

The overall problem is this. What are we looking for? Are we mining the system or farming it? If we are looking for ways to pay for health care it is one thing. If we are looking for more and better healthcare it is another.

Mining the System

If we are looking for more ways to pay for health care we are on the wrong track to begin with. Paying for something is not the same thing as getting what you are paying for. We have been attempting to pay more to get more health care, but with a monopoly situation it doesn't work that way.

Whether the allegations are true or not, there is a charge that Senator Diane Feinstein has arranged for her husband to earn the brokerage fees for selling government property that will net him 950 million dollars. This charge would indicate mining the system. Representative Pelosi has been alleged to have allowed her husband to obtain government contracts. If this allegation is true this amounts to the same thing. The result of mining the system is in an imbalance of the economy. It places all the resources of the economy in the hands of a few people. These people can never have enough objectives to use all of their resources. At the same time, people who need these resources to contribute to society are unable to make their contribution because they do not have those resources.

Those who are concerned about getting more money for healthcare are typically mining the system..

Farming the System

There is a difference between mining and farming. Mining takes what is there are puts it into use. Since it deals only with what is already there, eventually the thing being mined will run out. Ghost towns dot the landscape in Nevada. These are towns that grew up around a source of silver ore. When the lode ran out the townspeople left. The town died.

We need to farm the system. A Farmer uses what is there, but they add what is needed to get a good crop. If the soil is deficient in nitrogen, he adds fertilizer. If the rainwater erodes the soil he ditches and channels it. We need to farm the healthcare system. The result of farming the healthcare system is more healthcare. The result of mining the healthcare system is more cost and less healthcare.

We Need to Invest in our Healthcare Workers

It takes a lot of time and effort to become a good doctor. We should be proud that these people who care for other's health should be free of the costs of becoming a physician. One suggestion would be to buy all the costs of the education from the student and his lenders, and amortize that cost over a period of years, possibly twenty years. This could be paid by the physician, but it would be better to forgive this debt at 5% each year if he remained fulltime, maintaining an office in the profession for a rate of at least 1800 hours per year, during that time.

By removing the pressure of debt from the student's shoulders, and providing a solution to the problem of educational debt, the life of the physician would be immensely improved.

At the same time, we would need to insist that the physician would remain in general practice for a period without taking on a specialty. Certain specialties, such as gynecology or pediatrics, which have a workload that rivals general practice could be exempted but specialties that have little demand would require that the specialist would also be a general practitioner. The same requirement would apply to research and development

More Bang for the buck

We invest heavily in preparing our healthcare providers. That investment makes our physicians capable of providing the healthcare we need. When we allow these well trained physicians to earn enough to cut their work time to less than the time that full time employee has to work in order to make a living, we are wasting our investment. The short answer to this problem is to say that we will not include them in the Medicare system unless they maintain their office at a rate of 40 hours a week. This computes to 2080 hours per year, but holidays are 40 hours and vacations are typically 80. Allowing 120 hours that cover unforeseen difficulties leaves us with 1800 hours per year. By requiring that a physician keeps working hours at a rate of 1800 hours per year would make a good return on our investment.

These hours would include professional education, and vacations when they are being calculated so that no elimination from the system for failing to maintain a proper work rate.

Research and Development

The government should not invest in research and development for diseases that affect only a few members of a population. This should not be prohibited, but such research and development should be funded by other sources and not the government. The healthcare needs of the general population should be paramount. A disease that affects only one person in 100.000 should be set aside while those health problems that affect most of the population are taken care of. Even in the parable of the lost sheep, when the shepherd went out to find the lost lamb, he left the 99 safely in the fold, where they were safe. It is important to deal with the common diseases before we spend time and money on the rare ones.

Legal Problems Malpractice

No trial for malpractice should be considered legitimate if there is no peer of the doctor or other health care professional on the jury. According to the Magna Carta, all legal trails should be held with a jury of one's peers. Amendment VI to the Constitution endorses the requirement that all legal processes require an impartial jury. This requirement that a jury of one's peers demands that juries include at least one person of equal knowledge and standing has been allowed to lapse. Until the judiciary is forced to recognize the need for fair representation on the jury, the legal situation of physicians is analogous to enabling the fox to guard the henhouse.

Medical Patents

All patents that are essential to the health and or safety of the individual should be made perpetual to allow for the production of the medicine by as many producers as is possible. Instead of monopoly that now provides a return on the efforts of the researcher, a license amounting to 4% of manufactures pricing or 1 % of retail pricing would be required of all producers, whether they were involved in the research needed or not.

Set Prices

Doctors have told me that Health care cannot work with set prices for diagnoses. They use as an example anew bionic knee that cost more than the old one. This argument is specious. First the research to make the new knee is a diversion from the provision of patient care, but more importantly because the new knee would be a separate diagnosis, and could be priced differently.

The use of set pricing is essential in monopoly situations. If the monopoly sets the price itself, it will set it as high as possible. As essential as electricity is, the price of that electricity would be at the mercy of the electric company if it was not regulated. Since all health services are monopolies, the same rationality should be invoked to hold prices in line with value. As each region of the country has a different hospital system, that regulation should be handled regionally. For that purpose, a regional board of price management should be developed in each region, to place a price on each diagnosis in the book of diagnoses The board should have representatives of health care professionals, the government, and the public, so that each can be heard about each diagnosis.

Payment to licensees only

The problem that arises when anyone can bill Medicare and get paid immediately should be met by using a list of those who can bill Medicare. That list is available by using the identification on the list of licensed health professionals, and the authority under which the license was issued.

The problem of unauthorized individuals billing the system is a political one. People who bill Medicare without proper authorization are mining the system and contributing nothing to our health care services. By requiring that the billing physician or other healthcare professional identifies himself this waste of money can be reduced.

Of course there are items that can promote health that are provided by non-licensed. Here it would be well to remember the difference between general contractors and subcontractors. The general contractor deals with the customer. For the subcontractor the general contractor is the customer. If the item needed for the health of the patient is provided by a nonlicensed vendor, the subcontractor can bill the doctor and the doctor can put in the claim.

Incomplete Claims

Claims requesting payment by Medicare should be complete. To be complete, there are many items that should be on the claim for payment. An incomplete claim should be returned to the claimant and not accepted for payment if incomplete. For example, the identification of the claimant should include the authority issuing the license under which the health professional is licensed and the licensee's identification on that authority's list.

Additionally, the invoice should identify every item used in the treatment of the patient. This means that there will be a brand, a name of the product used, a quantity, and a price. Of course there will be items that are to minimal to count, such as three tissues, or amount of lotion used on the patient, but the majority of items used, whether by number or by value, should be listed on the invoice. Any failure to provide this information would mean that the invoice would be returned as incomplete and require completion before the claim could be processed.

One of the items that should not be overlooked is the name and contact information for the patient or responsible party. This would allow Medicare to verify with the patient that the claim was valid.

Avoid Sidetracking New Physicians

Before a newly licensed healthcare worker specializes, or transfers to research and development he needs to provide healthcare to the general public for a period of time. That time could be short such as two years, but having spent the costs of the physician's education Medicare should insist that it get the services it has paid for by buying the costs of that cost of education. To accomplish this, the money due for reimbursement of those educational costs would not be forgiven when the doctor chooses to specialize during those early years.

Specializing in pediatrics or gynecology is just as necessary as general practitioners. Such specialties should be exempt from this requirement, but a specialty that has few patients should be delayed for a time.

Hospital Independence

Hospitals are "non-profit businesses." The money that they earn has been used to fund other businesses. One business that has been linked to hospitals has been healthcare insurance. This linkage is a conflict of interest. The hospital is tempted to not accept any insurance other than its own, and often refuses to accept such insurance. They are also inclined to use their reimbursement for healthcare services to enter other businesses such as real estate. They offer to rent offices to physicians and others, and magnify their profit by spending as much time on these businesses as they spend on healthcare.

The reimbursement for health services should be spent only on healthcare and the hospital should show that as much money as they have been reimbursed has been spent on care of patients.

Additionally, the separate businesses that the hospital finances should be managed separately, by a board that has no connection to the hospital. The need for the hospitals management should require fulltime management of the hospital, and not be distracted by the needs of the separate businesses.

Summary

The purpose of this book is to suggest that we need to have changes in our health care system. My wife and I were in Berlin. She took a shower. Unknown to her there was no hold bar on the side of the shower and in stepping out she fell. We went to the emergency room and she received a good clean up, 23 stitches and a tetanus shot- We had to pay the bill then, approximately $62. On telling a nurse after our return, the nurse replied that that would have cost $450 dollars in her emergency room.

When it is alleged that you can fly to Spain, have a knee replacement, spend a week on the beach and fly back for less than the cost of a knee replacement in the United States and realize that is true, you know that something is not being done right.

The suggested changes were listed above, but let me repeat them:

>Recognize that all personal services are monopolies, and regulate the prices allowed,
>Require that all payers pay the prices set by a representative board for each diagnosis,
>Pay only licensed health care providers at the address given on their license,
>Require juries to include at least one peer of the provider,
>Issue medically necessary patents to be in perpetuity with licenses to all qualified manufacturers

Eliminate cost plus pricing, require set prices,
Pay only to licensed healthcare providers,
Require full disclosure of all charges, by product, dosage, and all pertinent information,
Provide for subsequent audit, with patient verification,
Combine payments for specific treatments, allow contractor and subcontractor relations ships
Require full time provision of services to participate in Medicare reimbursement,
Eliminate negotiation of prices for insurance companies,
Require that the health care provider use reimbursement for health care
Buy student education costs and forgive as health care is provided,
Prevent specialization or research for early years of practice,
Recognize that medical care is not a matter of fear, but an attempt to care for the patient,
Separate non-medical business from health care provision

This has been a study of the healthcare situation in the United States at this time. The emphasis on mining the system rather than farming it has been and is a political matter. We need to review this situation and look closely at those politicians who have chosen to feather their own nest at the expense of the health of the people if this country.

I encourage all sensible people to look closely at this situation and encourage those who can to correct it.

www.ingramcontent.com/pod-product-compliance
Ingram Content Group UK Ltd.
Pitfield, Milton Keynes, MK11 3LW, UK
UKHW041413180426
11947UKWH00007B/102

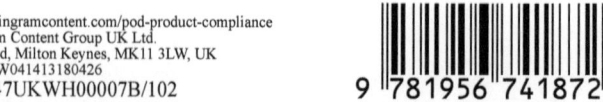